Book Title: **Dionn Fields Inc**

ISBN-13: 978-1499356984

ISBN-10: 1499356986

Title Page for: **Dionn Fields Inc**

The entire movies on paper studio productions, library was created By: Dionne L. Fields

Dionne L. Fields also made other contributions to this book title.

Illustrated

Photograph

Proofread

Editorial

Written

By Dionne Fields

1. Fields, Dionne. -Business 2.Woman Business Owner 3.African American Author Patients-United States-Biography. 4. Publisher/Entrepreneur.5. Movies On Paper Studio Productions.

6.Fields, Rain. 7. Ideas On Paper, 8. Sitcoms On Paper, Episode 1 and 10. Episode 2.

Book Title: **Dionn Fields Inc**

ISBN-13: 978-1499356984

ISBN-10: 1499356986

Movies on Paper Studio Productions Non – Fiction Children's Book Collection.

1.Rain's First Christmas, 2.Actor Rain, 3. Inventor Rain, 4. Super Model Rain, 5.God's Child One 6.Recording Artist Rain, and 7.Surfboarder Rain 8. Fashion Model Rain, 9. President Rain, 10. God's Child Two, 11.Ceo Rain, 12 Author Rain 13. Bully Proof Rain14.Rain Boy Fashion, 15. Football Team Rain, 16. Business Mogul Rain, 17. Pilot Rain, 18. Attorney Rain, 19. Rain's Children's Library, 20.Super Rain, 21. Philanthropist Rain, 22. Poet Rain 23.Rain Story Book Poem 24.Happy Mothers' Day.25. Rain Magical Library 26. Rain Fields Inc 27.Rain Retirement Party, 28.Sir Knight Rain Fields, 29. Rain Vacation 30. Rain' Famous Friends 31. Fireman Rain, 32. Prince Rain, 33. Musician Rain, 34. Fashion Designer Rain, 35. Cupcakes By Rain, 36. Astronaut Rain, 37. Photographer Rain, 38. Chef Rain, 39.Rain's Children's Book Museum, 40. Race Car Driver Rain, 41.The Rain Fields Children's book collection, 42, G.I.Rain

Movies on Paper Studio Productions Fiction Children's Book Collection.

1.BlueBerry Bed Time Story, 2. The Magic Cell Phone, 3.Red Rain Boots, 4. Bubble Bath Time, 5. Broccoli Meet Cheese, 6. Good Night Blanket, 7. The Lost Tooth, 8. Read Fairy, 9. **Sitcoms On Paper, Episode 1 and** 10.**Episode 2**

Movies on Paper Studio Productions Non- Fiction Novels.

1.Movies On Paper Studio, 2. mascara, 3. Honoring Colleges, 5. Documentary Of Real Champ, 6. Living For Today 7. September 11, 8. Sedreck Fields, 9.Greatness Endured 37 Losses, 10. Documentary Real Champ, 11. Sedreck Fields Scholarship Fund, 12. 10,000 Volunteer Hours, 13. No One Exempt From Hard Times, 14. National Book Signing, 15. Black History & Me, 16. 2012 By Dionne, 17. Theresita. 18. Unlimited God favor, 19. Black Movies On Paper, 20. Sedreck Fields Foundation, 21.Purpose & Reflections, 22. Behind Close Doors, 23.Facing Tomorrow 24. One Wish, 25. History Maker Nominee, 26. Dionne Fields Reality TV Show, 27. Cancer survival museum, 28. **Dionn Fields Inc**

Movies on Paper Studio Productions True - Crime Book Series.

1.The Untold Story, 2.Unpunished, 3. Whispering A Secret, 4.Pages Of Me Chapter One, 5. Pages Of Me Chapter Two, 6.Pages Of Me Chapter Three, 7. Pages Of Me Chapter Four, 8. Pages Of Me Chapter Five

Movies on Paper Studio Productions Ideas On Paper Book Series.

1.Re-designed Living Room Suite 2.Re-designed Light Weight Military Uniforms 3.Re-designed Toddler Strollers 4.Re-designed Ball Game Seats 5.Re-designed Lamps 6.Re-designed Bathroom Sets 7.Re-designed Business Chairs 8. Re-designed Car Seats, 9.Re-designed wall covers by :Mr.Diamond Fields

First published in the United States of America in 2014

By Dionne Fields (Publisher) new hardcover edition.

Library Of Congress Cataloging-In-Publications Data

Fields, Dionne L.

[Movies On Paper Studio Productions, Coming Soon To A Shelf Near You.]

Originally Published, 6331 Pleasant Ridge Rd. Knoxville, Tennessee.37921

Library Of Congress Control Number:

ISBN-13: 978-1499356984

ISBN-10: 1499356986

http://theresit.webs.com/

https://www.facebook.com/dionnfieldsinc

This novel is written & created By Dionne Fields

Printed in the United States of America May 1, 2014

Content Page

Movies On Paper Studio Productions

Book Title: **Dionn Fields Inc**

Introduction by, Dionne Fields

Introduction page

Complete Book Title

Book Title: **Dionn Fields Inc**

The complete story behind.

Dionn Fields Inc

Dionn Fields Inc.

The story about Dionn Fields Inc.

Its my goal to help woman fight Uterine Cancer.
To honor my mother's memory (Theresita Fields) 10-16-48 - 10-26-12.
And to raise funds for a new facilty in Atlanta
near the Cancer Center of America.

Mission

My mother had Uterine Cancer.There was very little resourse to help my mother,
with her battle of Uterine Cancer. I want to help one million women, fight for
the cure of Uterine cancer. Uterine Cancer support group,survivor resources
resourse for,medicine,personal care items,wigs,food,ect.

Biography

Read for the cure, I have books for sale to raise funds to
fight against Uterine Cancer.
I began writing novels after a career as a self-published author
and after publishing a dozen short stories.
http://www.onlineslibrary.webs.com/

Company Overview

My mission is to save lives and stop uterine cancer forever.
To also provide supportive services to woman impacted by a diagnosis of
Uterine cancer. Your support will help give anyone facing
Uterine cancer a place to turn for answers and help

Description

The fight to cure uterine cancer and to raise funds for a new facilty in Atlanta,
near the cancer center of america.
To provide the resourse
and the support for women, who has been diagnose with uterine cancer.

General Information

To provide assistance during the lowest point for women battling uterine cancer.
To partner with local community health charities to
offer women free to low cost yearly exams and pap smears.

A Daughter's Tears

I started working on a personal journal the very day; my mother was diagnose with uterine cancer.

Each day, that I visit her, I would take notes of her daily progress.
Once she is in remission of her cancer, I will publish this journal into a self help novel at my online book store and library.

http://www.onlineslibrary.webs.com/

This new self help novel title a daughter Tears, will help daughters of ages cope with having a parent, who is dying with any type of cancer.

I have started an online cancer support group for daughters, who moms are fighting Uterine Cancer.

I pray that my experience with my mother, would help another daughter survives this painful, sleepless ,emotional , heart retching tragic , that I'm dealing with alone each and every day.

http://theresit.webs.com/
In my spare time when, I'm unable to sleep at night, I would work on my magazine called: Cancer & Answers.

A health magazine about cancer.

And also resource articles to help cancer patients, with help & support to make their fight against cancer much easier to fight. In my new magazine,

I will feature the survival story of the month.

I believe God for the Funding to launch this new cancer magazine this year.

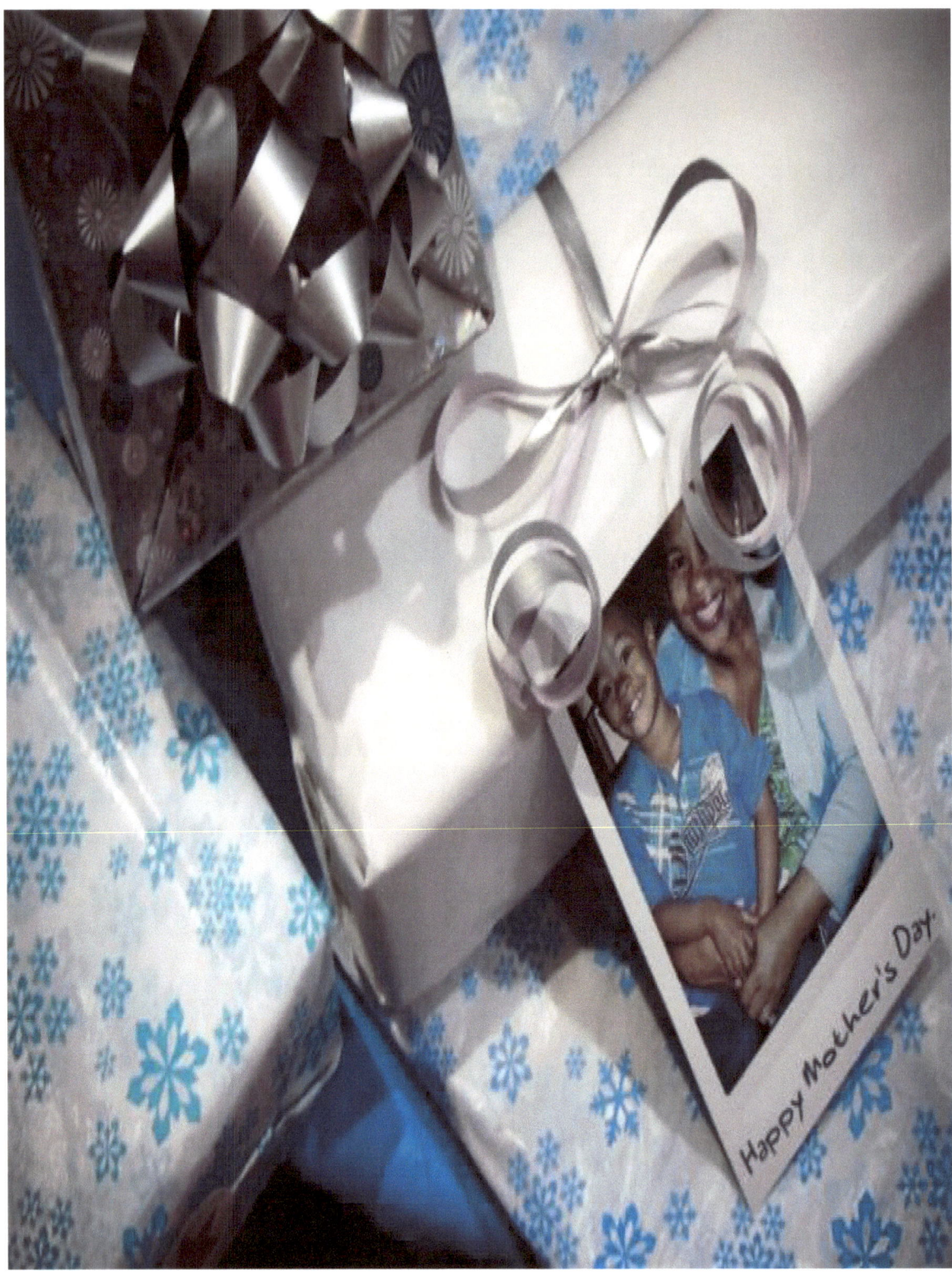

The Gift

I'm working on raising money to purchase a building, to have the Gift program in honor of my mother's memories.

The Gift program will help other women like my mother, during their treatments of Uterine Cancer.

The gift program will provide 5 free panties and 2 free bras plus free personal hygiene items.

And when funding is available, free robe with matching sleepers.

The Gift will be in my mother's memories, because my mother was my special Gift from God.

How you can help.

Local business owners, to sponsor this monthly event, to fight against uterine cancer
Local florist to donate flowers, to women who just been diagnose with uterine cancer.

Local bakery to donate bakes goods, for our monthly bake sale and cake walk for the kids.

Local hotel to donate personal hygiene wash clothes and towels, the will help women diagnose with uterine cancer, feel fresh and clean during daily cancer treatment and hospital visits.

Volunteers to make get –well cards for all the women, who just been diagnose with uterine cancer.

Local artist or band to donate their talent to our monthly benefit concerts on Saturday, from 1-3pm.

Local Radio station and radio personality to have a radio thon, to help us fight against uterine cancer.

The community to donate non perishable items and can goods to our weekly food pantry, to help women diagnose with uterine cancer with children.

Uterine cancer survivals to come share their stories, to encourage other women during our weekly uterine cancer support group.

Thursdays 6-8pm a drawing for a gift basket at each meeting.

Founder of the Gift Program. Dionne Fields

Pink Suede and Pearls is a new organization designed to uplift and promote positive self esteem to woman undergoing treatment for breast, ovarian, **uterine**, or other **"female" cancers** and survivors of those diseases.

Our official fragrance will be Avon's Pink Suede.

We will have an annual fund raiser in the Chicago area but the main focus of this group is to take small feminine gifts to women undergoing cancer treatment at least once per year all across the USA.

Gifts must include a faux pearl pair of earrings or other piece of jewelry.

Thanks inadvance for helping my mom fight Uterine Cancer.

Ms. PSAPS Atlanta Princess 2007

Dionne Fields

http://psaps.tripod.com/id2.html

Local artist or band to donate their talent to our monthly benefit concerts on Saturday, from 1-3pm.

Local Radio station and radio personality to have a radio thon, to help us fight against uterine cancer.

The community to donate non perishable items and can goods to our weekly food pantry, to help women diagnose with uterine cancer with children.

Uterine cancer survivals to come share their stories, to encourage other women during our weekly uterine cancer support group,

Thursdays 6-8pm a drawing for a gift basket at each meeting.

Founder of the Gift Program. By Dionne Fields

A Costly Disease Uterine cancer is associated with significant costs which impact on the affected individuals and their families, as well as society.

[1] The costs of Uterine cancer include those which relate directly to medical care, such as the costs of drugs and physician services, and also indirect costs which include costs associated with loss of productivity e.g. lost or decreased ability to work ect..

Cancer Survival Museum for women.

Sponsor By Dionn Fields Inc

Goal: $250000.00 | Raised: $0.00

Started: May 4, 2014

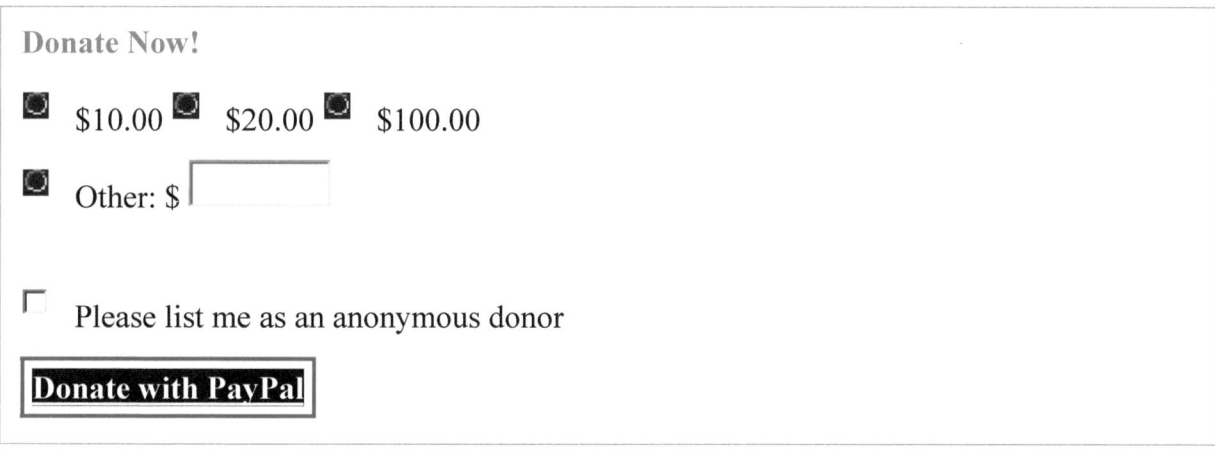

Cancer survivor museum for women diagnose with uterine cancer, ovarian cancer, cervical cancer.

This museum is in honor of my mother Theresita Fields.

She was diagnose with uterine cancer in 2012 and lost her fight just 10 days of her 64th birthday on October 26, 2012.

Thereista fields 10-16-48- 10 26-12.

To honor your love one, in the cancer survival museum.

If you would like to honor your love one, by adding them to our cancer survival museum you can honor them today with your contribution of $99 per person.

Today's special for a limited time is only $49 per person.

All the funds raise from your contribution will be use to purchase a building in the Atlanta, Georgia area.

You will receive an invitation to our grand opening once we purchase the cancer survival museum.

Your love one name will all be feature inside the museum as well.

1.Theresita Fields 10-16-48 --- 10-26-12 Uterine Cancer - $99

2.Your love one Uterine cancer or ovarian cancer or cervical cancer-$49
Pay pal.com

sender : k21mr8@yahoo.com

Amount $49

Dionn Fields Inc

Raising Funds to save lifes.

Goal: $15000.00 | Raised: $0.00

Started: May 3, 2014

Ends: May 4, 2014

It's my goal to help woman fight Uterine Cancer.
To honor my mother's memory (Theresita Fields) 10-16-48 - 10-26-12.

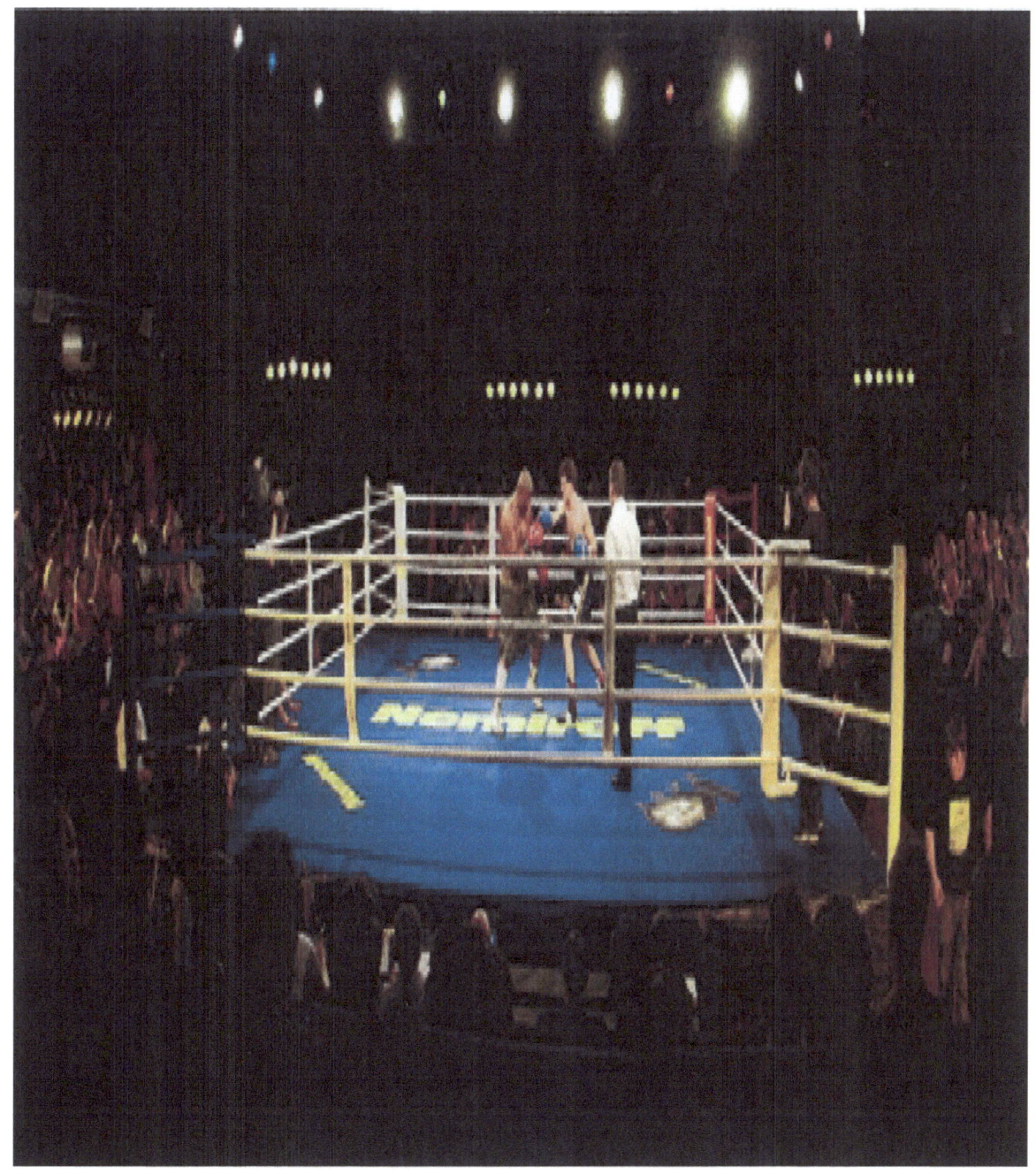

My mother was diagnosing with uterine cancer in 2012.

In her memory, we will be fighting for her to save lives and to end the disease of uterine cancer.

The funds raised will be used to purchase a new facility for our organization.

To participate in this event, to fight against uterine cancer.

Team #1 pink with pink gloves is fighters.

Team #2 black with black gloves are uterine cancer.

The event is fighting against uterine cancer.3 rounds for 3 minutes each fight.

You may fight for a love one who has been diagnoses with uterine cancer.

(Fighters)And you can help find a cure for uterine cancer.

(Uterine cancer) Kids ages 5-10 cost to participate is only $10.00 each.

Boys against boys

Girls against girls

Fight time 5:00pm

Youths ages 11-14 cost to participate is only $10.00 each.

Fight time 6:00pm

Teens ages 14-17 cost to participate is only $10.00 each.

Fight time 7:00pm

Adults ages 18 and over cost to participate is only $20.00 each.

Group cost to fight a team of 6 is just $60.00 .

Business cost to fight a team of 6 is just $60.00 .

Fight time 8:00pm.

Register today, before all the seats and fights are sold out.

Tickets at the door to attend our fight night event.

Adult tickets just $10.00,

Kids tickets just $5.00

 free under 3 years old.

Advance tickets purchase on line is only $7.00 Adults, (ages 18 and up)

Advance tickets purchase on line are only $5.00 kids(ages 5-17)

Advance tickets purchase online are only $30.00 per (Group and Business Teams)

You may purchase The Theresita Fields story her battle against Uterine Cancer today:

http://www.lulu.com/shop/dionne-fields/the-untold-story/paperback/product-20516453.html

Just bring copy of book to the event to be autograph with your receipt.

And your admission is free!

Volunteers are needed to be ring girls.

Volunteers are needed to be referee.

Volunteers are needed to set up boxing ring.

Volunteers are needed to hand out flyer.

Volunteers are need to video record the event.

Volunteers are needed to take photos.

Business who would like to cater this event, please email me today. Jesus1st2me@yahoo.com

The boxing gym location in Atlanta will be announced soon.

(TBA) Friday June 8, 2013

Sponsorship for this event are welcome.

Follow link below to register and purchase advance tickets.

To pay login into paypal account.

http://www.paypal.com/

To send money enter k21mr8@yahoo.com

Add amont and subject.

EXAMPLE

Advance tickets for fighting on pink team.

Advance tickets for fighting on black team.

Advance ticket to attend fight night.

Read For A Cure Campaign.

Our goal is to sell one million books, to help one million women diagnose with Uterine Cancer.

For every book purchase,all proceeds will help save lives and raise funds for a new facaility in Atlanta.

1.http://www.lulu.com/shop/dionne-fields/the-untold-story/paperback/product-20516453.html

2. http://www.lulu.com/shop/dionne-fields/theresita/paperback/product-20453355.html

The fight against uterine cancer, still continues.

Thanks mom, for always believing in me, and for buying me 1st novel.

Thanks mom for making me a better mother to my kids.

You are the reason I'm where im at today and thank you.

I love You Mom!!

Your Daughter (Dionne)

Walk for the cure.

We will be walking at local bike trails and parks.

Our walk for the cure will also begin with a picnic.

Walk for a cure will be once a month on saturday mornings.

between 10 am and 12 noon.

Sponsors are welcome to support this event.

Volunteers are need to hand out bottle water.

Volunteers are need to set up pic nic tables.

Volunteers are need to place pink and white ballons on bike trail and in the park.

To participate in this event is only $10 per person at the door.

And kids under the age of 18 is only $5 per child.

Mothers with strollers are $1.00.

Door prizes and free food will be given away.

To sign up or volunteer and even sponsor this event.

The Fight Against Uterine Cancer.

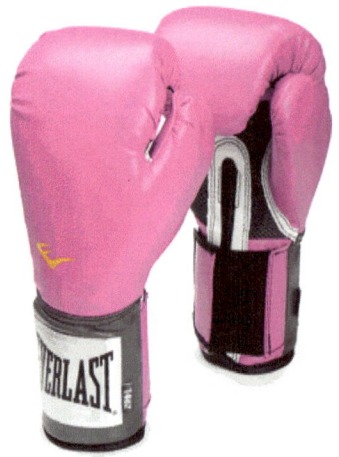

We will be having ongoing events to raise fund, to fight against Uterine cancer.

And to purchase a new facalitiy in Atlanta,Georgia.

To be near the new Cancer Center Of America.

Its my goal to honor my mothers memory, by help miilions of diagnose with uterine cancer.

Month | Week | Day | **All Events**

Date	Time	Event
Fri. 5/11	5:00 PM	Friday Night Fights [IMAGE] My mother was diagnosing with uterine cancer in 2012. In her memory, we will be fighting for her to save lives and to end the disease of uterine cancer. The funds raised will be used to purchase a new facility for our organization.
Sat. 5/16	10:00 AM	Walk for the cure [IMAGE] We will be walking at local bike trails and parks. Our walk for the cure will also begin with a picnic. Walk for a cure will be once a month on saturday mornings. between 10 am and 12 noon. Sponsors are welcome to support this event.
Thu. 5/22	6:00 PM	Uterine Cancer Support Group. [IMAGE] Uterine cancer survivals to come share their stories, to encourage other women during our weekly uterine cancer support group. Thursdays 6-8pm a drawing for a gift basket at each meeting. The community to donate non perishable items.

Fri. 5/23	1:00 PM	music concert for the cure A music concert for the cure. sponsors are welcome to help with this event. Gospel music and praise and worship music is perferable. Local artist or band to donate their talent to our monthly benefit concerts on Saturday, from 1-3pm .
Fri. 6/13	5:00 PM	Friday Night Fights [IMAGE] My mother was diagnosing with uterine cancer in 2012. In her memory, we will be fighting for her to save lives and to end the disease of uterine cancer. The funds raised will be used to purchase a new facility for our organization.
Sat. 6/21	10:00 AM	Walk for the cure [IMAGE] We will be walking at local bike trails and parks. Our walk for the cure will also begin with a picnic. Walk for a cure will be once a month on saturday mornings. between 10 am and 12 noon. Sponsors are welcome to support this event.
Thu. 6/26	6:00 PM	Uterine Cancer Support Group. [IMAGE] Uterine cancer survivals to come share their stories, to encourage other women during our weekly uterine cancer support group. Thursdays 6-8pm a drawing for a gift basket at each meeting. The community to donate non perishable items .
Fri. 6/27	1:00 PM	music concert for the cure A music concert for the cure. sponsors are welcome to help with this event. Gospel music and praise and worship music is perferable. Local artist or band to donate their talent to our monthly benefit concerts on Saturday, from 1-3pm
Fri. 7/11	5:00 PM	Friday Night Fights [IMAGE] My mother was diagnosing with uterine cancer in 2012. In her memory, we will be fighting for her to save lives and to end the disease of uterine cancer. The funds raised will be used to purchase a new facility for our organization.
Fri. 8/8	5:00 PM	Friday Night Fights [IMAGE] My mother was diagnosing with uterine cancer in 2012. In her memory, we will be fighting for her to save lives and to end the disease of uterine cancer. The funds raised will be used to purchase a new facility for our organization.

Theresita Memories.

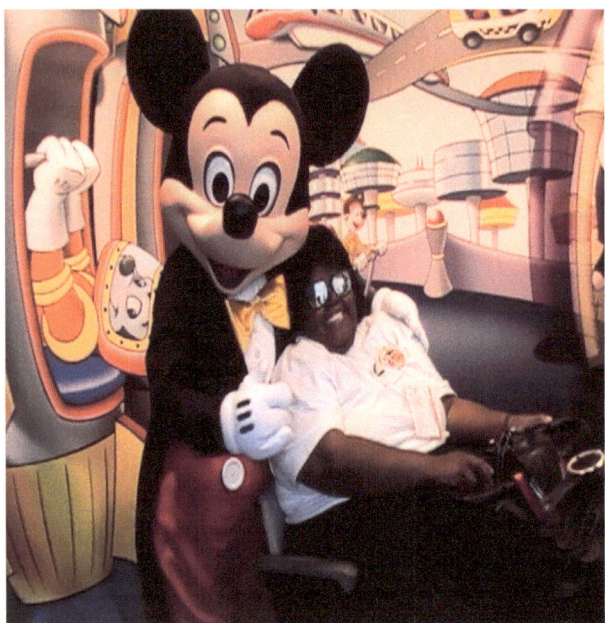

Diagnosis: Uterine cancer

"To take her family to Orlando"

Although Theresita has had a life rich with love, she has never had the financial means to provide her family many extras.

Now faced with a limited prognosis in her battle with uterine cancer, she knows her time is limited, and wishes more than ever for the opportunity to be the type of grandmother she's always wished she could be.

Theresita's dream is to take her daughter and grandchildren to Orlando; it would be their first family vacation.

"Every day I suffer, I go through my cancer treatments and they are painful," she says. "I go through life watching people I love suffer because they take care of me every day.

I just want a chance to do something special for them.

I want to be the grandma who can give them presents and show my love. I've always wanted to give them a vacation and special memories.
" Theresita's family has begun saving in hopes their dream will soon come true; one grandson even sold his video game console for money to spend on Grandma during the trip.
Theresita's daughter adds, "Because of you we will be able to laugh and smile one last time."
http://www.dreamfoundation.org/dreams/theresita

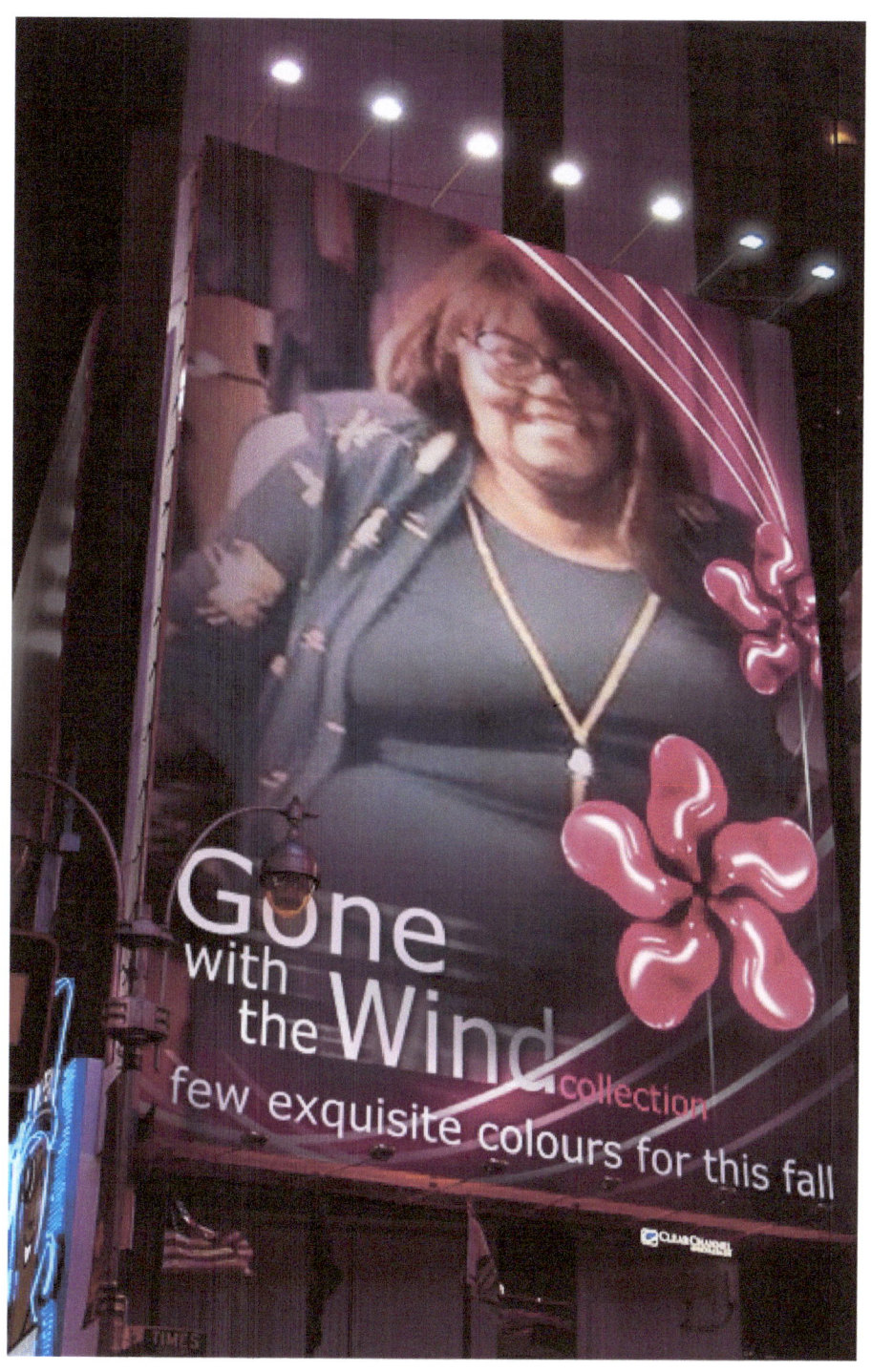

Just like the wind, my mother was Gone.

My mother use to weigh 410lbs , before she died she weighed only 287 lbs. I was so proud of her.

Patient Diagnosis	Date of Diagnosis	Cancer Stage	Status	Died
Uterine Cancer	05/16/2012	4	radiational	10/26/12

Cancer Survival Museum for women.

Cancer survivor museum for women diagnose with uterine cancer, ovarian cancer, cervical cancer.

This museum is in honor of my mother Theresita Fields.

She was diagnose with uterine cancer in 2012 and lost her fight just 10 days of her 64th birthday on October 26, 2012.

Thereista fields 10-16-48- 10 26-12.

It's my goal to help woman fight Uterine Cancer.

To honor my mother's memory (Theresita Fields) 10-16-48 - 10-26-12.

And to raise funds for a new facility in Atlanta

near the Cancer Center of America.

My mother had Uterine Cancer.

There was very little resource to help my mother,
with her battle of Uterine Cancer.

I want to help one million women, fight for
the cure of uterine cancer.

Uterine Cancer support group, survivor resources
resource for, medicine, personal care items, wigs, food, ECT.

Uterine Cancer Support Group.

Uterine cancer survivals to come share their stories, to encourage other women during our weekly uterine cancer support group, Thursdays 6-8pm a drawing for a gift basket at each meeting.

The community to donate non perishable items and can goods to our weekly food pantry, to help women diagnose with uterine cancer with children.

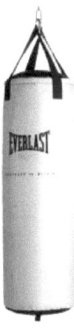

We also have a punching bag and gloves for women diagnose with uterine cancer. To fight the bag to release stress and fears. And to knock out uterine cancer.

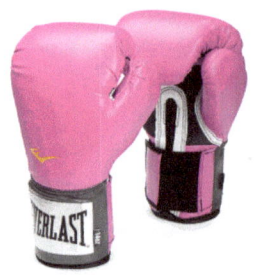

To participate in knock out uterine cancer is only,$5.00 for every 10 minutes.

This is a wonderful event to raise funds and to have fun.

Theresita Fields Story,since christmas 2010.

My mother has complain about severe abdominal pains,nausea and vomitting.

An agressive tumor,was found mothers day 2012.

In October 2012 she lost her fight against uterine cancer.

I lost two people that day, my mom and my best friend.

http://www.lulu.com/shop/dionne-fields/the-untold-story/paperback/product-20516453.html

Cancer Tears

In Loving Memory Of Theresita Fields.October 16,1948- October 26, 2012.

 We will miss you!! It's a different kind of war, that I have to fight each day.

When the enemy is Uterine Cancer.

When fighting runs in my blood, I have to win this fight for my family.

 Im bless to have the blood line of one of america's great generals.

And as his great grand daughter ,Im honor to fight with all my heart.

http://www.lulu.com/shop/dionne-fields/the-cancer-tears/paperback/product-20516570.html

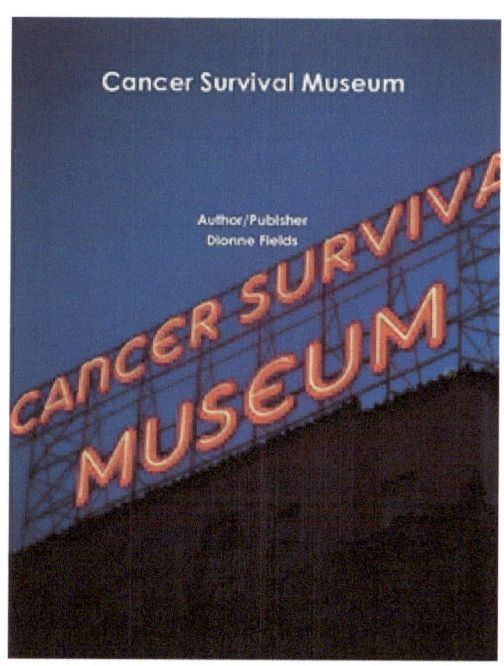

Cancer survivor museum for women diagnose with uterine cancer, ovarian cancer, cervical cancer.

This museum is in honor of my mother Theresita Fields.

She was diagnose with uterine cancer in 2012 and lost her fight just 10 days of her 64th birthday on October 26, 2012.

Thereista fields 10-16-48- 10 26-12

DEPARTMENT OF THE TREASURY
INTERNAL REVENUE SERVICE
PHILADELPHIA PA   19255

DATE OF THIS NOTICE: JU 12 2002
NUMBER OF THIS NOTICE: CP 575 E
EMPLOYER IDENTIFICATION NUMBER: 33-1016167
FORM: SS-4
0532639511 0

FOR ASSISTANCE CALL US AT:
1-800-829-1040

DIONN FIELDS INC
% DIONNE L FIELDS
PO BOX 1267
NORCROSS GA   30091

OR WRITE TO THE ADDRESS
SHOWN AT THE TOP LEFT.

IF YOU WRITE, ATTACH THE
STUB OF THIS NOTICE.

WE ASSIGNED YOU AN EMPLOYER IDENTIFICATION NUMBER (EIN)

Thank you for your Form SS-4, Application for Employer Identification Number
(EIN). We assigned you EIN 33-1016167. This EIN will identify your business account,
tax returns, and documents, even if you have no employees. Please keep this notice in
your permanent records.

Use your complete name and EIN shown above on all federal tax forms, payments and
related correspondence. If you use any variation in your name or EIN, it may cause
a delay in processing and incorrect information in your account. It also could cause
you to be assigned more than one EIN.

If you want to apply to receive a ruling or a determination letter recognizing
your organization as tax exempt, and have not already done so, you should file Form
1023/1024, Application for Recognition of Exemption, with the IRS Ohio Key District
Office. Publication 557, Tax Exempt Status for Your Organization, is available at
most IRS offices and has details on how you can apply .

MAY 1, 2000
Keep this part for your records.   CP 575 E (Rev. 1-20

THIS CERTIFICATE IS TO BE POSTED IN A CONSPICUOUS PLACE IN THE BUSINESS HEREIN DESCRIBED.

BUSINESS CERTIFICATE

AUGUSTA

THIS CERTIFICATE EXPIRES

2003

ACCOUNT   2003#029702

ISSUE DATE   08/08/2003

CERTIFICATE ISSUED IN NAME OF

DIONN FIELDS INC.

Wednesday, December 31, 2003

Yearly

08/08/2003-12/31/2003

SIC CODE   813910

BUSINESS CATEGORY   BUS ASSCO

BUSINESS TYPE SERVICE

DIONNE FIELDS

In August 2000, Fields founded Dionn Fields, Inc.— the umbrella organization for a number of programs that work to help homeless women and children, including My Homeless Child. Fields also operates Home Safe, a program that finds homes for homeless women and their children.

THE LICENSE AND INSPECTION DEPARTMENT SHALL HAVE THE RIGHT TO SUSPEND ANY CERTIFICATE IF THE BUSINESS VIOLATES ANY LAW OR ORDINANCE OF THE UNITED STATES, THE STATE OF GEORGIA, OR RICHMOND COUNTY.

ORIGINAL   45229

AUGUSTA

2004

BUSINESS CERTIFICATE

THIS CERTIFICATE EXPIRES

Friday, December 31, 2004

Yearly

01/01/2004-12/31/2004

ACCOUNT   2004#029702

ISSUE DATE   09/16/2004

CERTIFICATE ISSUED IN NAME OF

DIONN FIELDS INC.

SIC CODE   813910

BUSINESS CATEGORY   BUS ASSCO

BUSINESS TYPE   SERVICE

BUSINESS LOCATION

1333 BLOUNT AVE

CERTIFICATE ADDRESS INFORMATION

DIONNE FIELDS

DIONNE FIELDS

JEFF

GEORGIA

MAILING ADDRESS INFORMATION

DIONNE FIELDS INC

THE LICENSE AND INSPECTION DEPARTMENT SHALL HAVE THE RIGHT TO SUSPEND ANY CERTIFICATE IF THE BUSINESS VIOLATES ANY LAW OR ORDINANCE OF THE UNITED STATES, THE STATE OF GEORGIA, OR RICHMOND COUNTY.

ORIGINAL   55519

THIS CERTIFICATE IS TO BE POSTED IN A CONSPICUOUS PLACE IN THE BUSINESS HEREIN DESCRIBED.

BUSINESS CERTIFICATE

AUGUSTA

2005

THIS CERTIFICATE EXPIRES

Saturday, December 31, 2005

Yearly

01/01/2005-12/31/2005

ACCOUNT	2005#029702
ISSUE DATE	01/27/2005

CERTIFICATE ISSUED IN NAME OF
DIONN FIELDS INC.

SIC CODE	813910
BUSINESS CATEGORY	BUS ASSCO
BUSINESS TYPE	SERVICE

BUSINESS LOCATION

1333 BLOUNT AVE

CERTIFICATE ADDRESS INFORMATION

DIONNE FIELDS

DIONNE FIELDS

1736

GEORGIA

MAILING ADDRESS INFORMATION

DIONNE FIELDS INC

THE LICENSE AND INSPECTION DEPARTMENT SHALL HAVE THE RIGHT TO SUSPEND ANY CERTIFICATE IF THE BUSINESS VIOLATES ANY LAW OR ORDINANCE OF THE UNITED STATES, THE STATE OF GEORGIA, OR RICHMOND COUNTY.

COPY   57521

31

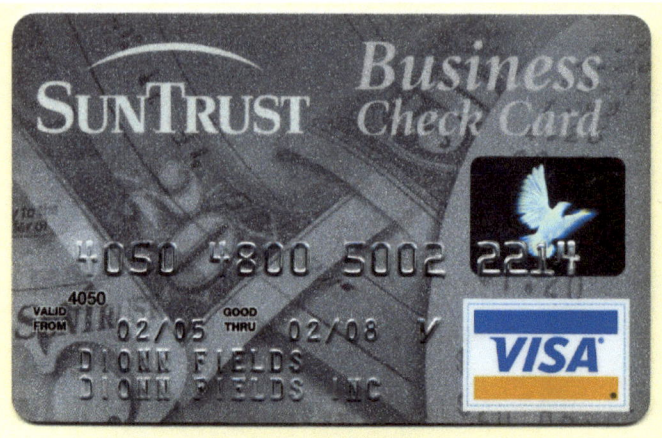

DIONN FIELDS INC 10/2002   770-566-0111   1013
PO BOX 1267
NORCROSS, GA 30091-1267   64-10/610 ★

33-1016167

_____
                                                         DATE

PAY TO THE
ORDER OF _____   VOID _____

                                                    DOLLARS 🔒 Security
                                                                  Features
                                                                  Details on
                                                                  Back.

SunTrust
SunTrust Bank

FOR _____   _____ MP

⑆061000104⑆1000006129539⑈ 1013 ⑇0000000300⑇

© HARLAND 2001

DISIASTER VOLUNTEERS OF GHANA

Ms Dionne Fields Children Nation Tour.

PROGRAMME OF ACTION.

8th March 2003.

Meeting with Youths and Children at Ho.

- *Drummer.*
- *Launching/Fundraising of Dionne Fields Children Computer Shelter Ghana.*
- *Give away to children.*

9th March 2003.

Church Service.

- *Visit Sunday school Children.*
- *Meet the entire congregation and raised fund.*

Project Site Visit – 1.

- *Ho Community Girls Training Center (HCGTC).*
- *Amedzofe.*

13th March 2003.

Mother Tear Project.

- *Visit to mothers who lost a son or daughter due to illness.*
- *Courtesy call on Chief and Elders of Ho traditional area.*

14th March 2003.

Project Site Visit – 2.

- *Visit to disadvantage children at Kpotoe, Dzofe, and Akuatey.*

Review of the visit to Ghana.

- *General Meeting.*

From: "yinkah richard" <ryinkah@hotmail.com> | **This is Spam** | **Add to Address Book**

To: d10nn@yahoo.com

Subject: Important Message from the Children!

Date: Tue, 07 Jan 2003 20:37:58 +0000

Dear Dionne,
How are you today? Hope you are doing supper as we are also doing towards
your coming. By the close of the week we will have a final confirmation from
the all the people who you will meet during your 5 days visit to
Ghana. Now
the children will be very happy if you can extend to at least 10 days which
you will have a personal time to meet the rest from the other parts of the
Ghana..
Now we have set up a fundraising children's to raise fund both at the local
and international level towards your coming, which will help to meet the
cost of some things here. Because the press, media, hotel (5 star),
conferences room, and also you will be interviewed on the national
televison, and some pettey expenses, we need to get some funds to pay in
advance to meet this project and that the children are appealing to all, to
join hand in this.
We will be so much happy if you can let , concern philanthropists,
individuals , churches among others to help in this fundraising
.Please
send the first two pages of your passport as an attachment to us too, all
this will help in meeting the officials we need to be part of the program, I
have been able to get you the handset, and you will have access to internet
everyday. A laptop at you disposal.
Please let us join hand in this as soon as we can.
Thanks a million for your support for the children and they are waiting to
meet you soon.

This message is not flagged. [Flag Message - Mark as Unread]

From: "yinkah richard" <ryinkah@hotmail.com> | **This is Spam** | **Add to Address Book**

To: d10nn@yahoo.com

Subject: Message from Ghana

Date: Fri, 10 Jan 2003 10:40:32 +0000

Dear Dionne,
Thanks for the reply and hope this finds you well. I have been out
countryside to meet some youths and children for a community
development
initiative at the rural level.
What's the news there?
With us here everything is fine and all we doing from now till you
is
to put everything in place.
I will send you a final program activity as soon as we have finish
on
it so that you will also prepare yourself with it. We want to make
coming one of the greatest one on the continent that is why we doin
all we
can to make the children/youths/mothers and the people of Ghana kno
you
presences.
With meeting the children and youths you will about 5,000 ✗
children/youths in
the capital of Ghana and then over 100 at the rural level for which
will
come from schools, village home, shelters, churches among others. A
with
the mothers you will also meet over 100 so all this are the work we
doing
towards your coming to be a memorable one as Ghana is the gateway t
Africa.
As I said we will send you a final program list as soon as it is in
hand.
Also in the program list, we are trying to see if you can meet the
president
of Ghana or the vice president apart from meeting the minister for

yinkah richard <ryinkah@hotmail.com> wrote:

> Dear Dionne,
> Thnaks from the children of Ghana for the respone and they wish to see you
> on day on project here in Ghana. they are waiting for your welcome
> package.Please send it to the address below and they hope to get it as soon
> as they can and will share it with other children around the community.
> The address is:
> Care for Children
> Disaster Volunteers of Ghana
> P.O. BOX H814
> HO VOLTA REGION GHANA
> PHONE;+233-24-734074
> Please inform us as soon as you send it.
> All the best and hope to hear from you soon.
> Richard Yinkah

36

The Secretary of State
of the United States of America
hereby requests all whom it may concern to permit the citizen/
national of the United States named herein to pass
without delay or hindrance and in case of need to
give all lawful aid and protection.

Le Secrétaire d'Etat
des Etats-Unis d'Amérique
prie par les présentes toutes autorités compétentes de laisser passer
le citoyen ou ressortissant des Etats-Unis titulaire du présent passeport,
sans délai ni difficulté et, en cas de besoin, de lui accorder
toute aide et protection légitimes.

SIGNATURE OF BEARER/SIGNATURE DU TITULAIRE

NOT VALID UNTIL SIGNED

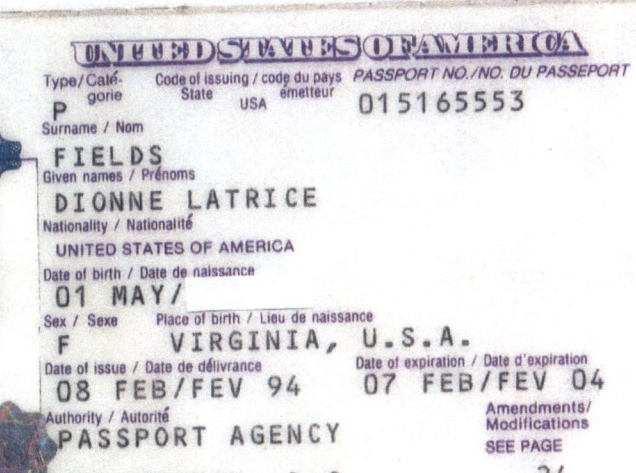

UNITED STATES OF AMERICA

PASSPORT / PASSEPORT		

Type/Caté-gorie: P

Code of issuing / code du pays State USA émetteur

PASSPORT NO./NO: DU PASSEPORT
015165553

Surname / Nom
FIELDS

Given names / Prénoms
DIONNE LATRICE

Nationality / Nationalité
UNITED STATES OF AMERICA

Date of birth / Date de naissance
01 MAY/

Sex / Sexe
F

Place of birth / Lieu de naissance
VIRGINIA, U.S.A.

Date of issue / Date de délivrance
08 FEB/FEV 94

Date of expiration / Date d'expiration
07 FEB/FEV 04

Authority / Autorité
PASSPORT AGENCY

WASHINGTON, D.C.

Amendments/Modifications
SEE PAGE
24

P<USAFIELDS<<DIONNE
0151655531USA7005015F0402073<<<<<<<<<<<<<<0

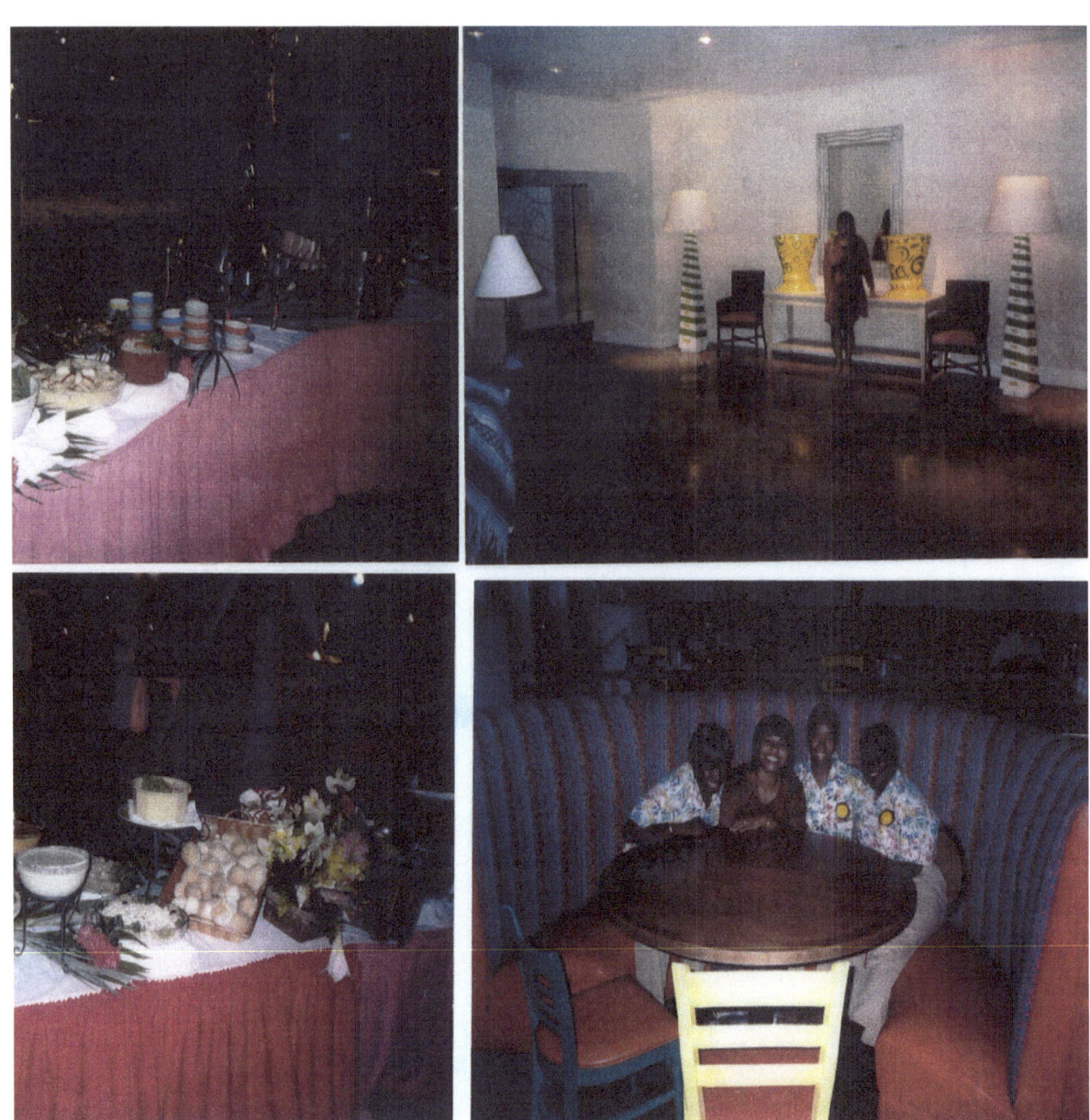

Area Women Making A Big Difference In The Lives Of Others

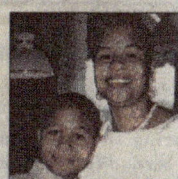

From Personal Trauma, Fields Triumphs To Help Others In Similar Situation

BY KATE WICKER

AUGUSTA—With over 3,000 volunteers across 50 states and 36 countries, Dionne Fields, founder of My Homeless Child, is touching the lives of thousands of homeless children by remembering their birthdays.

But to say My Homeless Child had humble beginnings doesn't even come close to describing how one woman transformed a difficult situation into an opportunity to make a difference.

Gwen Pinkerton of Norcross, Ga., is one of Field's many volunteers who helps reach out to homeless children by providing birthday cakes, candles and birthday gifts.

"Programs like this are essential to our community. These children are our future,

and they need to know that there are people who care about them. I can't imagine what a child goes through being homeless or being in

Birthday parties for homeless kids among services offer through the organization

a shelter due to neglect or abuse," Pinkerton said.

Fields cannot only imagine it—she lived it.

Fields and her son, Diamond, lived on the streets out of a car for three years.

"My son didn't ask to be homeless. I can remember my son waking up on the streets and the sadness I felt," she says.

Like some four million other women in the U.S., Fields was a victim of domestic abuse. In 2000, she was living in Virginia working to suppport her son while living in fear and torment. When the court issued a restraining order against her former fiance, he "hired" stalkers to follow Fields everywhere she went.

"People would follow me to work and follow Diamond when he went to school. They would threaten and harrass us. I was scared for myself and for my son," she recalled.

After more than two years of abuse and harrassment, Fields decided it was time to leave.

She also began to explore the idea of starting her own nonprofit.

"You have a lot of time to think when you're homeless. I couldn't sleep at night. I'd watch over Diamond, and that's when I started thinking and writing about My Homeless Child. I knew I wanted to reach out to other women and children who were homeless or victims of abuse."

With no money or resources, Fields turned her idea that came to her during sleepless nights into a burgeoning nonprofit.

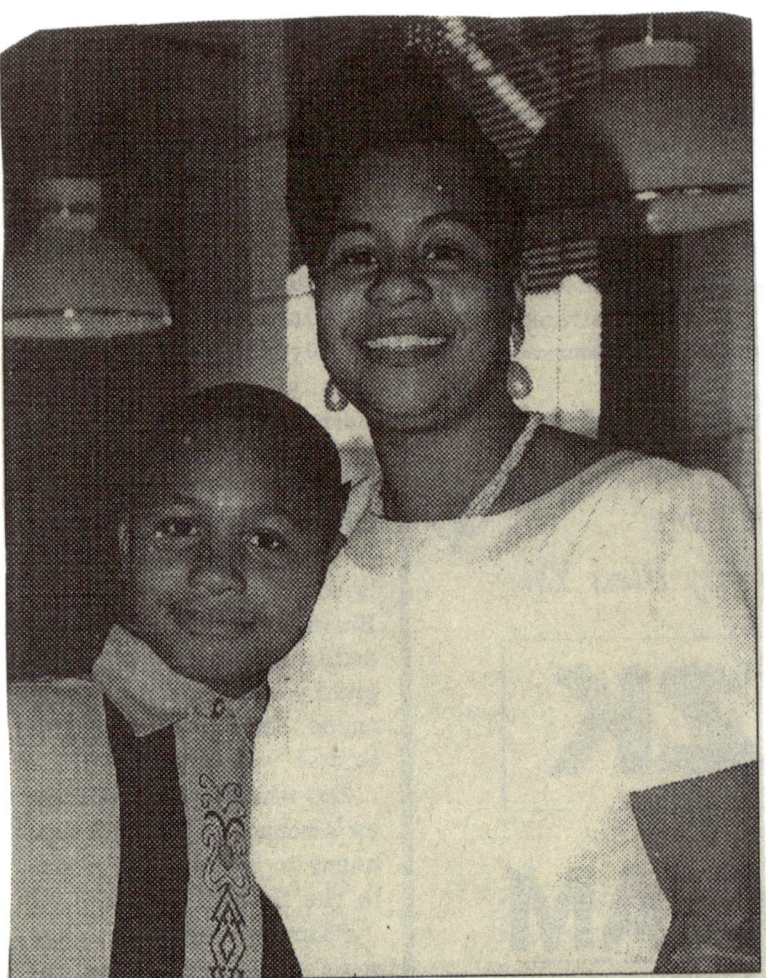

DIONNE FIELDS, pictured with son Diamond, wants to make a difference for those mothers and children who have to endure the "heartbreaking" homelessness she and her son experienced.

"I tried to go to abuse and homeless shelters, but they were all filled," she remembers. "I knew we had to get away from the abuse, but we didn't have anywhere to go. I didn't have family to turn to, and despite the court's orders, my abuser or his stalkers were everywhere we went."

Fields finally quit her job and used her savings to move to Georgia. The only home she and her son had was a car, but Fields was determined to restore hope in her life. She would send Diamond to school after cleaning him up with baby wipes. While he was away, Fields spent long

"When we were homeless, Diamond spent three birthdays with no gifts, no presents. I couldn't stop thinking about how I didn't want any other children to suffer the way he did," she says.

"I wanted to figure out how we could get out of the situation and never go back. I'd work out of the trunk of my car. I'd go to agencies like United Way and talk to them about my program. I researched how to get nonprofit status from the government. And I did all of this for Diamond. My son gave me the drive to move forward."

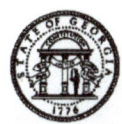

STATE OF GEORGIA
OFFICE OF THE GOVERNOR
ATLANTA 30334-0900

Sonny Perdue
GOVERNOR

April 8, 2003

Ms. Dionne Fields
3530 Ashford Dunwoody Rd. #229
Atlanta, GA. 30319

Dear Ms. Fields:

I regret the delay in my reply to your correspondence received during the transition period of my administration. Please be assured that this in no way diminishes its importance to me.

It must be a source of great pride to own four nonprofit organizations, and I am pleased to commend you for such resourcefulness. You have my best wishes for continued success.

Sincerely,

Sonny Perdue

SP:pm

This message is not flagged. [Flag Message - Mark as Unread]

Date: Tue, 27 May 2003 16:20:02 -0400
From: "Governor Mark Sanford" <Governor@govoepp.state.sc.us> | **This is spam** | **Add to Address Book**
To: myhomelesschild@yahoo.com
Subject: Your Correspondence

May 27, 2003

TO: Ms. Dionne Fields
        myhomelesschild@yahoo.com

Dear Dionne,

Thank you for your e-mail. Your work for the homeless in our state is to be commended.
Through your acts of volunteerism, you have exhibited the finest qualities of servant leadership. Thank you for your continued hard work
Take care.

Mark

National Spokes Woman for the Homeless Children.
Dionne Fields

April 13,2008

My Resources

National Service
Briefing

Service News

Press Releases

Dionne Fields

Home Page

General Motors

2008 SPONSOR

PRESENTING

SPONSOR

National Youth

Service Day

April 11,17 2008

By:Michelle Littleton   Date:03/24/2000 - 12/31/2009

It brings me great Honor to Represent the Homeless Children all around the world. No child in America ask to be Homeless neither did my son Diamond. For three long years my son and I have been homeless living on the streets and in my car for three years due to Domestic Violence. Today Im able to remeber all the homeless children in a shelter or on the streets on their birthday with a birthday cake and birthday card. From May 2000-March 2003 was the times my son and I have been Homeless. We still don't own Our own home as of yet but we are not sleeping in my car or own the streets. I still believe God that one day soon I will have the Keys to our very own place. Until then I will continue to support all the Homeless Children in America:

Dionn Fields Inc

Originally published:
02 /24 /2008

Related link: http://www.onlineslibrary.webs.com

Point of Contact: (865) 207-8274

Content Provided by: Dionne Fields

THE WHITE HOUSE

WASHINGTON

July 29, 2002

Dear Ms. Fields:

The President asked me to thank you for your letter inviting him to the Young Boys and Girls Athletic Sports Fundraiser/Book Signing in Atlanta, Georgia, on August 17, 2002. Although the President is appreciative of the support your invitation represents, it is with sincere regret that we must decline the invitation.

Unfortunately, as the schedule for the next few months has developed, we have had to make some difficult decisions. I do not foresee an opportunity to add this event to the calendar. I know this response comes as a disappointment. However, I want to assure you that your letter received every consideration.

The President asked that I take this opportunity to thank you for your letter. Please know that your comments and suggestions are always welcomed.

Sincerely,

Bradley A. Blakeman
Deputy Assistant to the President
and Director of Appointments and Scheduling

Ms. Dionne L. Fields
Young Boys and Girls Athletic
Post Office Box 1267
Norcross, Georgia 30091-1267

U.S. OFFICE OF PERSONNEL MANAGEMENT

Paul T. Conway
Chief of Staff White House

Office of the Director
1900 E Street, NW Room 5H09
Washington, DC 20415

Telephone: 202-606-1000
Fax: 202-606-2183
Email: pconway@opm.gov

HECTOR V. BARRETO
ADMINISTRATOR

U.S. SMALL BUSINESS ADMINISTRATION
409 3RD STREET, S.W.
WASHINGTON, DC 20416

TEL: (202) 205-6605
FAX: (202) 205-6802

This message is not flagged. [Flag Message - Mark as Unread]

From: "Eldridge-Bailey, Adrienne - ETA" <Eldridge-Bailey.Adrienne@dol.gov> | **This is spam** | **Add to Address Book**
To: "'myhomelesschild@yahoo.com'" <myhomelesschild@yahoo.com>
CC: "Queen, Libby - ETA" <Queen.Libby@dol.gov>
Subject: RE: Area woman making a big Difference in the lives of others.
Date: Mon, 14 Jul 2003 14:31:40 -0400

Dear Ms. Fields:

This is in response to your e-mail message to Mr. Haskel Lowery volunteering the services of your organization to assist homeless women and children in communities throughout the country. Your message was forwarded to me for response.

We commend your courage and your efforts to reach out and assist homeless individuals who are often forgotten but are also the most in need of help. The activities of your organization appears to be a valuable resource that may be useful to constituents who are served by the U.S. Department of Labor's (DOL's) Employment and Training Administration workforce investment system.

You should know that under the Workforce Investment Act (WIA) of 1998, funds are provided to States and their local communities to provide a broad array of employment and training activities and continued supportive services for eligible young people and adults. Since states and local areas have primary responsibility for managing youth programs under WIA, you may be interested in contacting the local workforce investment area office for possible funding assistance and information. The contact person is:

Mr. Patricia Sermon
818 Pollard Boulevard, SW
Atlanta, GA 30315-1523
Telephone: (404) 658-9675

If you are interested in contacting other local workforce investment offices, a listing of the local WIA offices can be found on the National Association of Counties (NACO) website at: http://www.naco.org/Template.cfm?Section=Workforce_Development&Template=/cffiles/wia/wia_srch.cfm. Once at NACO's website you must click on a state in order to locate a specific local WIA office.

I hope this information is helpful.

Sincerely,

ADRIENNE ELDRIDGE
Workforce Development Specialist
Office of Youth Services

Every businesswoman survival tools.

I want to help every woman who, has a dream of starting a business.

Even if you have been thinking about owning your own business.

Through faith and prayer anything is possible.

After reading this novel my personal story with my company.

Through my experience this book will, inspire you.

To triumph during you're most difficult times, with limited resources and support.

I have had great joy in sharing with every woman my personal experience through hard times and struggles made me depend on God more now than ever before.

My faith in my lord and savior Jesus Christ has been the one thing that kept me going.

 The only thing that will help you survive the hard times as a business owner will be your faith and trust in God.

A daily prayer before each morning you start your business will help you in so many ways.

Example:

Dear, Heavenly Father

Thank you for blessing me with the wisdom and knowledge to trust you to help me

Run this business of faith with guidance.

I will trust you to pour favor upon my business

To bring people my way to be a blessing.

Amen.

Business Mothers

My new project targeted for women with children who has or wants to start their very own home base business.

For almost 10 years movies on paper studio productions has been my home base business.

I'm now spending quality time with my sons.

I'm very happy about being an author writing self-help books and children books from home with my kids.

I encourage people all across America to support business mothers who works from home so they can take care of their children and earn an income.

There are so many talented business mothers who works from home from baking, sewing, making candles, writing screen plays and poetry ect.

We are in
need of a
building.   Building Fund

Dates: May 02, 2014 - December 02, 2014
Location: 3535 Peachtree RD NE suite 520-539, Atlanta, Georgia, 30326,
United States
Organization: Dionn Fields Inc
Website: http://theresit.webs.com/

Area of Focus: Children and Youth,
Community Development,
Community Service and Volunteering,
Economic Development, Family and
Parenting, Foundations, Fundraising,
and Philanthropy, Human Services,
Multi-Service Community Agency,
Poverty and Hunger, Social Enterprise
and Economic Development, Sports,
Recreation, and Leisure, Travel and
Transportation

Campaign posted on: May 2, 2014
Phone: 404-276-5849
Language(s): English
Contact person: Dionne Fields

Description:

Our organization needs a building.
Our non-profit organization needs a building in Atlanta, Georgia.
The building will be use to help women with children each day.
Our family food pantry and close closet.
And many other services like Christmas toys give away and back to school
drive.
We will be serving all 9 counties in Atlanta Area.
Our athletic youth program will also help young athletes.
Our uniform closet, sports equipment room, and snack room, athletic gear and
shoe room.
We will be helping hundreds of woman and children in the community each
day and thousands each week.
With your support in a building we can rebuild our Atlanta community during
these touch times in this recession.
Why should our children and youth have to suffer during these hard times?

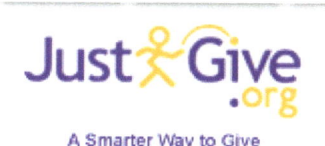

A Smarter Way to Give

Dionn Fields Inc

3535 Peachtree RD NE

Suite 520-539
Atlanta, GA 30326

GENERAL INFORMATION

Contact: Ms. Dionne Fields, Owner/CEO

Telephone: (404) 276-5849

Fax: (404) 442-8831

E-mail: jesus1st2me@yahoo.com

Web Site: www.onlineslibrary.webs.com

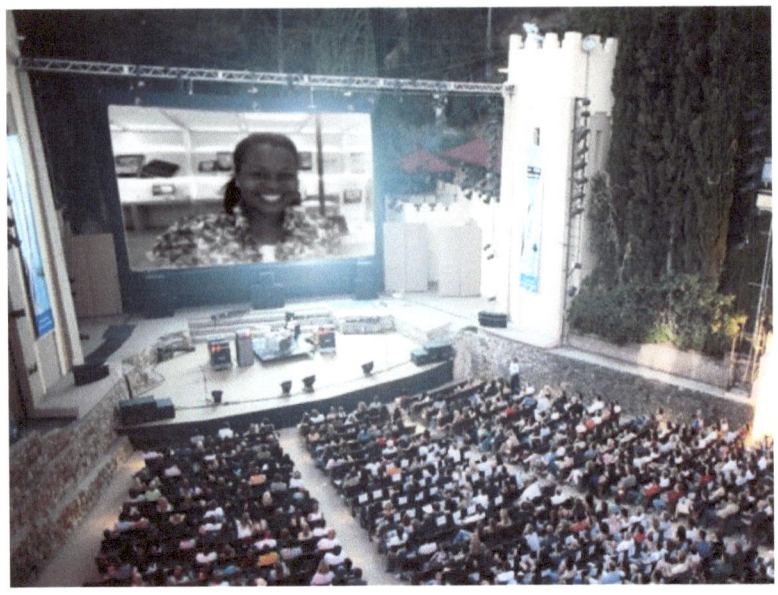

Dionne Fields bases Dionne Fields Reality TV show, on the novel of the same name.

Since December 1999, I have been volunteering over 10,000 volunteer hours.

This is a true story base on my life as a nonprofit business owner.

I have been blessing, with the opportunity of working with some of our amazing volunteers all across America.

Dionne Fields Reality TV show will feature silent Heroes, of women, men and children.

These are the silent hero's of America, who volunteer each day.

It's my dream to honor the volunteers who have supported my organization for a decade.

To have a major television network, see behind the scene of people volunteering, each day in our community.

This would inspire a major movement for charities all around the world.

Order your very own copy today at:

Dionne Fields Reality TV show (book) limited Edition

http://www.lulu.com/content/7842512

*Writers Guild of America # 1455427

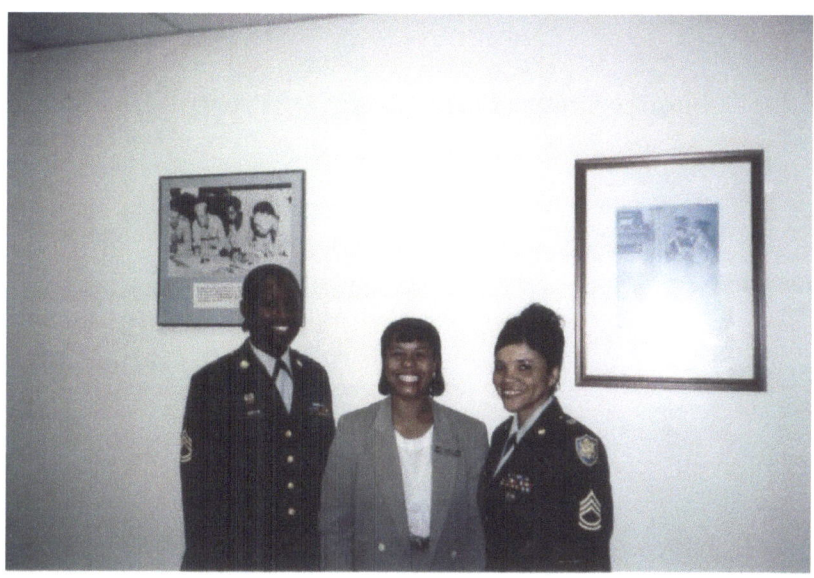

10, 000 volunteer hours

I started from December 1999- December 2000 my volunteer hours would have been 20-25 hours a week.

About 80-100 volunteers hours. A month when there was 5 weeks in a month.

 A grand total of 1, 200 Hours.

Un paid hours went to working, researching, getting my 501(c) 3 from the IRS, computer time on getting other volunteers to help, letting them know their assignments each week, sending out volunteer welcome packages, making up volunteer training material, making copies each day, Administration work, networking chamber of commerce, food pantry, New programs services and creating volunteer opportunities, fund raising.

Online communicating with volunteers all across the globe through email. Spokes woman for the homeless, Ect.

1. December 1999-December 2000 volunteer hours that year my 1st year in Business was 1,2000.

 Every Time I breathe - For every child who mother or father has passed away, we send each child and inspirational card from the heart.

2.December 2000-December 2001 volunteer hours that year my 2nd year in Business was 1,2000.

Get-Well wishes - We mail out hundreds of get-well cards to critical ill children at all the Ronald Mc Donald House Charities.

3.December 2001-December 2002 volunteer hours that year my 3rd year in Business was 1,2000.

. My Homeless Child - We make birthday cards and birthday cakes to all the homeless children in a shelter on their birthdays.

4.December 2002-December 2003 volunteer hours that year my 4th year in Business was 1,2000.

A Mothers Tears - We send hundreds of encoring poems and purple ribbons to mothers all around the world who has lost a son or daughter due to death or illness, military war.

5.December 2003-December 2004 total volunteer hours that year my 5th year in Business was 1,2000.

. Love worth waiting for - We send hundreds of encoring poetry and white ribbons to all the mothers around the world who has a child still missing.

6.December 2004-December 2005 total volunteer hours that year my 6th year in Business was 1,2000.

Send A Prayer - We have volunteers praying for people every 10 minutes each day for people who are in a crisis.

7.December 2005-December 2006 total volunteer hours that year my 7th year in Business was 1,2000.

Behind Close doors - We email hundreds of women who have been emotional abuse by family, friends, and co-workers. ect.

8.December 2006-December 2007 total volunteer hours my 8th year in business was 1, 2000

Sedreck Fields Foundation- Provides funding for youth athletes ages 4-18 with the funds they need to participate in sports.

9.December 2007-December 2008 total volunteer hours my 9th year in business was 1, 2000

Send A Hug - This volunteer opportunity is to honor all single moms who have raised a son alone. I take my hat off to each mother who had to be both parents to a male child alone. Send A Hug is a wonderful way to let mothers know all across the globe that being a single mom raising a male child is not easy. And we would like to send a hug cards today.

10.December 2008- 2009 are just bonus hours I stop counting my volunteer hours once I had reach a goal of 10,000.

Well you do the math 10 years x 1, 2000 an estimate total of 10, 000 volunteer hours.

11. December 2009- 2013 **total volunteer hours my 14th year in business was 15,000**

12. Today December 1999- 2014 is a grand total of 20,000 volunteer hours

10,000 Volunteer Hours was a goal I set for myself years ago.

When 1st started working at this wonderful non-profit organization.

I never thought I would have invested 10,000 volunteer hours.

Through blood, sweat, and tears helping so many people at just 1 hour at a time.

Community involvement helping others through volunteering those people is also called volunteer Heroes.

Big thanks to volunteermatch.org and Idealist.org.

They have some of the best volunteers in the world.

I hope this book encourage more people to volunteer and help in their community.

Purchase book at http://www.lulu.com/content/7426736

24-hour community food pantry and clothing closet in every major city in America to help rebuild America.

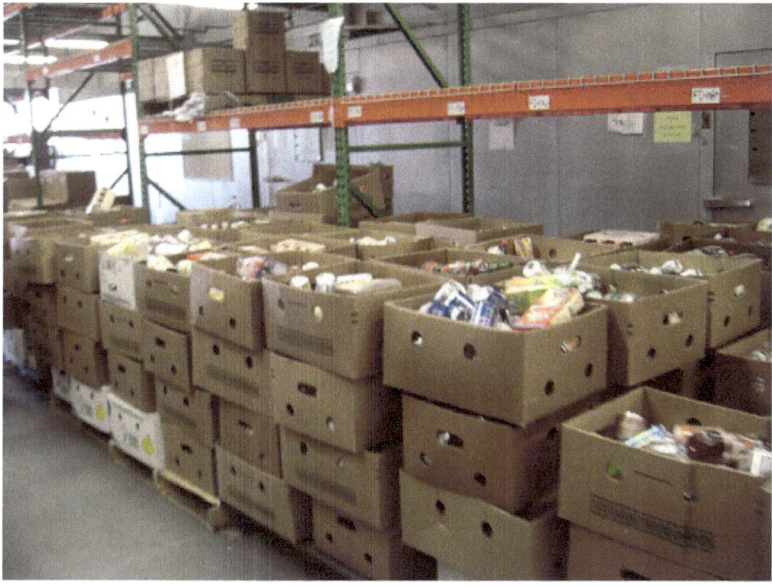

I'm just one woman who speaks on the behalf of millions of women with children, who can't help themselves.

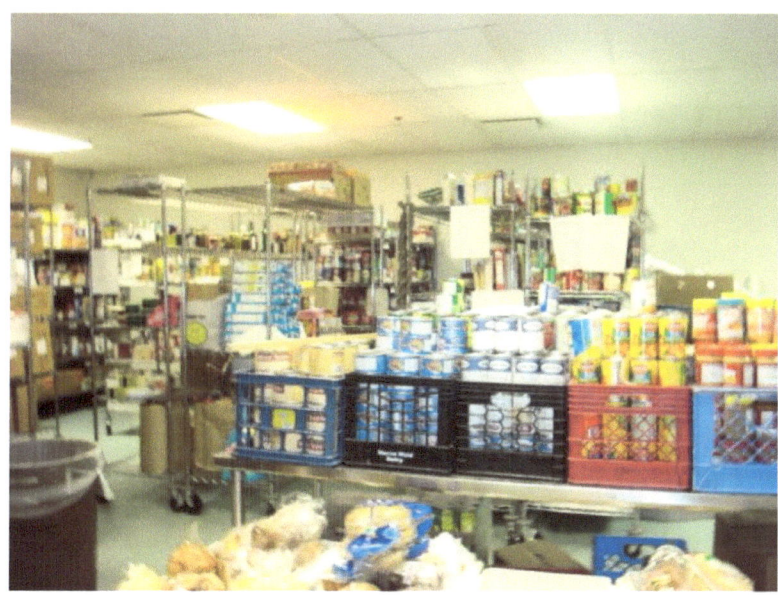

My passion and mission in this life is to open doors 24 hours a day 7 days a week.

To help women and children in need, for free food, free clothing, free emergency shelter, ect.

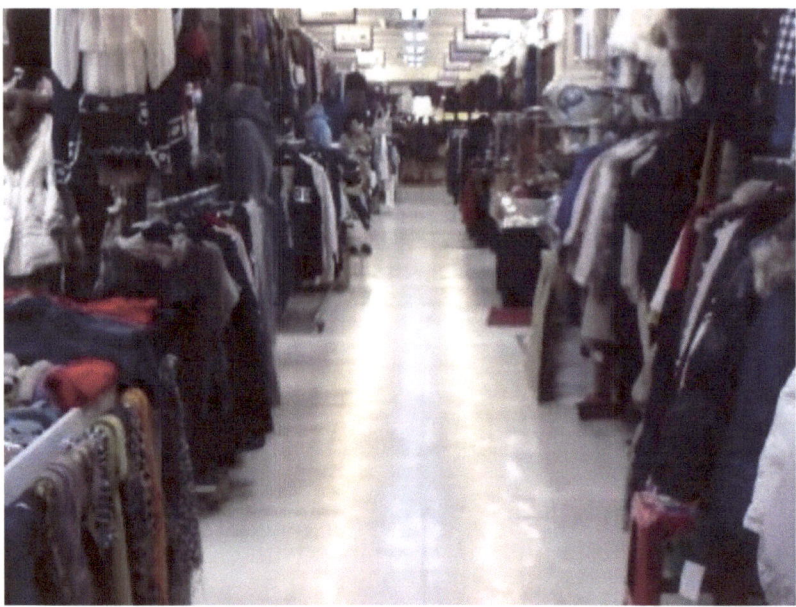

This would be the first 24-hour community family free food pantry & free clothing boutique for women with children in need.

Case by case basic, to survive the huge blow of this economy.
Those who read this story, pray that God would bless me with a building to continue this worthy cause.

Women with children who sustained losses, due to the economy, loss a job, tornado, flood, earthquake, or wildfire can begin applying for assistance today.

It is my prayer, to rebuild struggling families & community's one state at a time, working with Governors from each state.

There are so many ways that community groups and individual can help!

And this is why im selling my books to raise money for a building back in Atlanta, Georgia.

About the author.

I'm the author of, more than 50 book titles.

I began writing novels, after publishing a dozen short stories.

Movies on paper studio production, coming soon to a bookshelf near you.

When books & movies meet at the box office.

I enjoy business traveling, shopping for sales and playing golf.

And family vacations with my sons.

Dionn Fields Inc

This book is dedicated to my mother, who lost her fight against

Uterine cancer in 2012.

In memory of Theresita Fields October 16, 1948 – October 26, 2012.

http://theresit.webs.com/

The End

www.ingramcontent.com/pod-product-compliance
Lightning Source LLC
Chambersburg PA
CBHW050805180526
45159CB00004B/1553